C000172824

PLANT

BASED

DIET

RECIPES

DELICIOUS AND HEALTHY PLANT-BASED RECIPES FOR QUICK AND EASY MEALS

-CALLIE BLANTON-

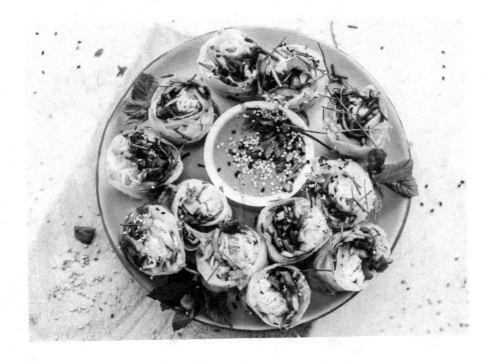

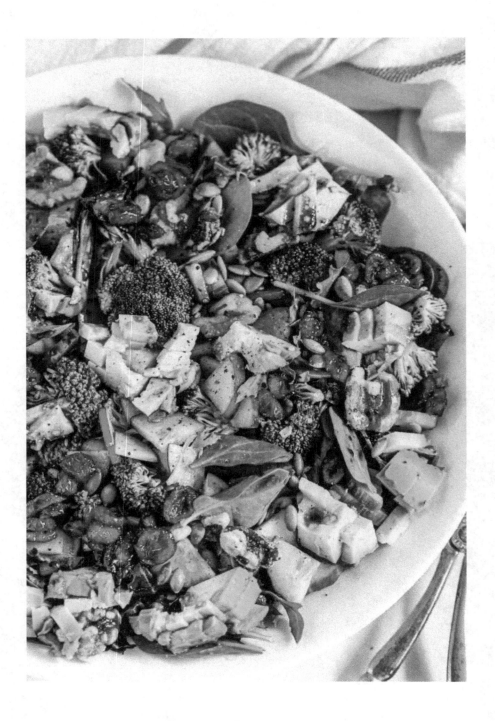

TABLE OF CONTENTS:

© Copyright 2021 by Callie Blanton All rights reserved.

The following Book is reproduced below with the goal of providing information that is as accurate and reliable as possible. Regardless, purchasing this Book can be seen as consent to the fact that both the publisher and the author of this book are in no way experts on the topics discussed within and that any recommendations or suggestions that are made herein are for entertainment purposes only. Professionals should be consulted as needed prior to undertaking any of the action endorsed herein.

This declaration is deemed fair and valid by both the American Bar Association and the Committee of Publishers Association and is legally binding throughout the United States.

Furthermore, the transmission, duplication, or reproduction of any of the following work including specific information will be considered an illegal act irrespective of if it is done electronically or in print. This extends to creating a secondary or tertiary copy of the work or a recorded copy and is only allowed with the express written consent from the Publisher. All additional right reserved.

The information in the following pages is broadly considered a truthful and accurate account of facts and as such, any inattention, use, or misuse of the information in question by the reader will render any resulting actions solely under their purview. There are no scenarios in which the publisher or the original author of this work can be in any fashion deemed liable for any hardship or damages that may befall them after undertaking information described herein.

Additionally, the information in the following pages is intended only for informational purposes and should thus be thought of as universal. As befitting its nature, it is presented without assurance regarding its prolonged validity or interim quality. Trademarks that are mentioned are done without written consent and can in no way be considered an endorsement from the trademark holder.

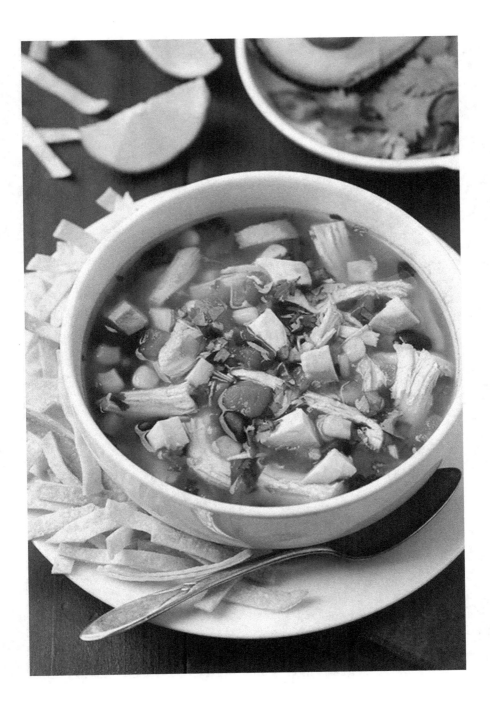

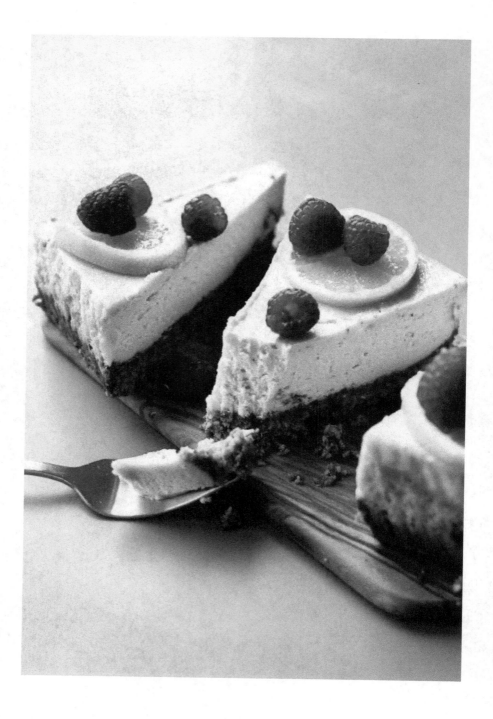

CHAPTER 1: **BREAKFAST RECIPES**

Pumpkin Pie Oatmeal

Prep:

10 mins

Cook:

35 mins

Total:

45 mins

Servings:

4

Yield:

4 servings

INGREDIENTS:

½ teaspoon vanilla extract

¼ teaspoon ground cinnamon

⅛ teaspoon ground ginger

¾ cup milk

5 tablespoons milk

1 tablespoon brown sugar

¼ teaspoon ground cinnamon

3 cups boiling water

1 cup steel-cut oats

1 cup pumpkin puree

DIRECTIONS:

1

Bring water to a boil in a saucepan; add oats, pumpkin puree, vanilla extract, 1/4 teaspoon, cinnamon, and ginger. Reduce heat to low and simmer, without stirring, until oatmeal is thickened, about 25 minutes.

2

Pour 3/4 cup milk into oatmeal, stir well, and cook for 10 minutes more. Spoon oatmeal into serving bowls and top with remaining 5 tablespoons milk, brown sugar, and 1/4 teaspoon cinnamon.

NUTRITION FACTS:

219 calories; protein 7.8g; carbohydrates 38.7g; fat 4g;

Breakfast Banana Green Smoothie

Prep:

5 mins

Total:

5 mins

Servings:

1

Yield:

1 serving

INGREDIENTS:

1 carrot, peeled and cut into large chunks

¾ cup plain fat-free Greek yogurt, or to taste

¾ cup ice

2 tablespoons honey

2 cups baby spinach leaves, or to taste

1 banana

DIRECTIONS:

1

Put spinach, banana, carrot, yogurt, ice, and honey in a blender; blend until smooth.

NUTRITION FACTS:

367 calories; protein 18.6g; carbohydrates 77.4g; fat 0.8g

Butternut Squash 'Porridge'

Prep:

10 mins

Cook:

50 mins

Total:

1 hr

Servings:

3

Yield:

3 servings

INGREDIENTS:

1 butternut squash, halved and seeded

water as needed

¼ cup coconut milk, or to taste

½ teaspoon ground cinnamon

1 tablespoon chopped walnuts

DIRECTIONS:

1

Preheat oven to 350 degrees F (175 degrees C).

2

Place butternut squash halves, cut-side up, in a baking dish; fill dish with 1/4 inch of water.

3

Bake in the preheated oven until softened, 50 to 60 minutes. Cool squash.

4

Scoop squash flesh into a bowl and mash with a fork or potato masher until smooth. Stir coconut milk and cinnamon into squash; top with walnuts.

NUTRITION FACTS:

242 calories; protein 4.9g; carbohydrates 49.9g; fat 6g;

Scrambled Tofu

Prep:

10 mins

Cook:

15 mins

Total:

25 mins

Servings:

4

Yield:

4 servings

INGREDIENTS:

ground turmeric to taste

salt and pepper to taste

½ cup shredded Cheddar cheese (Optional)

1 tablespoon olive oil

1 bunch green onions, chopped

1 (14.5 ounce) can peeled and diced tomatoes with juice

1 (12 ounce) package firm silken tofu, drained and mashed

DIRECTIONS:

1

Heat olive oil in a medium skillet over medium heat, and saute green onions until tender. Stir in tomatoes with juice and mashed tofu. Season with salt, pepper, and turmeric. Reduce heat, and simmer until heated through. Sprinkle with Cheddar cheese to serve.

NUTRITION FACTS:

190 calories; protein 12g; carbohydrates 9.7g; fat 11.5g;

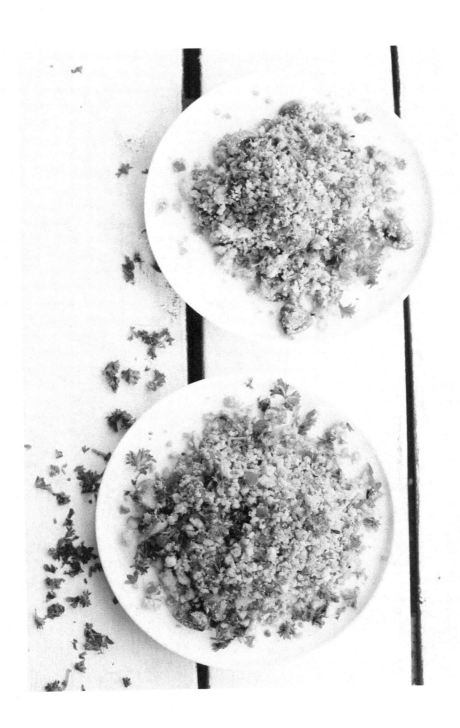

CHAPTER 2: **SOUP RECIPES**

Easy Cucumber-Dill Soup

Prep:

30 mins

Additional:

4 hrs

Total:

4 hrs 30 mins

Servings:

6

Yield:

6 servings

INGREDIENTS:

2 teaspoons white sugar

1 teaspoon garlic powder

1 teaspoon dried dill weed

1 teaspoon salt, or more to taste

1 teaspoon ground black pepper, or more to taste

4 large cucumbers - peeled, seeded, and cubed, divided

½ cup finely chopped yellow onion, divided

½ cup finely chopped celery, divided
½ cup grated carrots, divided
4 medium jalapeno peppers, seeded and finely chopped
¼ cup Greek yogurt
¼ cup sour cream

DIRECTIONS:

1

Set 1/4 cup of cubed cucumber aside.

2

Place remaining cucumbers, 1/4 cup onion, 1/4 cup celery, 1/4 cup carrots, jalapeno peppers, Greek yogurt, sour cream, sugar, garlic powder, dill, salt, and pepper into the bowl of an 8-cup electric blender or food processor and pulse until all ingredients are just blended.

3

Pour into a large bowl and stir in reserved 1/4 cup cucumber and remaining onion, celery, and carrots to add a little crunch to an otherwise creamy mixture. Taste for salt and pepper, adding more if desired.

4

Place into the refrigerator for at least 4 hours before serving.

NUTRITION FACTS:

82 calories; protein 2.6g; carbohydrates 12.8g; fat 3.2g; cholesterol 6.1mg;

Mexican Rice Soup with Mushrooms

Prep:

20 mins

Cook:

35 mins

Additional:

15 mins

Total:

1 hr 10 mins

Servings:

4

Yield:

4 servings

INGREDIENTS:

¼ white onion

2 cloves garlic

1 (8 ounce) package sliced fresh mushrooms

2 jalapeno peppers, seeded and chopped

2 tablespoons chicken bouillon granules

2 cups hot water

1 cup uncooked white rice

1 tablespoon vegetable oil

4 cups water, divided

5 sprigs flat-leaf parsley

DIRECTIONS:

1

Combine hot water and rice in a bowl and soak for 15 minutes. Rinse until water runs clear and drain very well.

2

Heat oil in a saucepan over medium heat. Add rice and cook, stirring constantly, until translucent, about 5 minutes.

3

Combine 1 cup water, parsley, onion, and garlic in a blender. Process until smooth. Pour through a strainer into the saucepan with the rice and bring to a boil for 3 minutes. Add mushrooms and jalapeno peppers. Boil until slightly tender, about 2 minutes more.

4

Stir remaining 3 cups water and chicken bouillon into in the saucepan with the rice. Bring back to a boil, reduce heat, and cover. Simmer until rice is soft, about 15 minutes.

NUTRITION FACTS:

231 calories; protein 6.4g; carbohydrates 42.6g; fat 4.2g;

Tomato Basil Soup

Prep:

25 mins

Cook:

30 mins

Total:

55 mins

Servings:

8

Yield:

8 servings

INGREDIENTS:

1 (28 ounce) can tomato sauce

1 (8 ounce) can tomato sauce

1 ¼ cups chicken broth

2 tablespoons chopped fresh basil

1 tablespoon chopped fresh oregano

salt and ground black pepper to taste

1 ½ cups heavy whipping cream

6 tablespoons butter

1 onion, thinly sliced

15 baby carrots, thinly sliced

2 stalks celery, thinly sliced

3 cloves garlic, chopped

DIRECTIONS:

1

Melt butter in a large pot over medium-low heat; cook and stir onion, carrots, celery, and garlic until vegetables are tender, about 10 minutes. Stir in both amounts of tomato sauce, chicken broth, basil, and oregano. Increase heat to medium and simmer until soup is reduced, 10 to 20 minutes.

2

Pour soup into a blender no more than half full. Cover and hold lid down; pulse a few times before leaving on to blend. Add cream. Continue to puree in batches until smooth, transferring creamy soup to another pot.

3

Heat soup over medium-high heat until hot, about 5 minutes more.

NUTRITION FACTS:

270 calories; protein 3g; carbohydrates 10.1g; fat 25.4g;

Easy Ramen Soup

Prep:

10 mins

Cook:

27 mins

Total:

37 mins

Servings:

2

Yield:

2 bowls

INGREDIENTS:

2 egg yolks

¼ cup chopped scallions, or to taste

1 tablespoon soy sauce

1 cup kimchi

1 pound boneless chicken breasts

4 cups water

2 (3 ounce) packages ramen noodles (without flavor packet)

1 ½ cups frozen peas and carrots

DIRECTIONS:

1

Bring a pot of water to a boil; cook chicken until no longer pink in the center, 15 to 20 minutes. An instant-read thermometer inserted into the center should read at least 165 degrees F (74 degrees C). Drain water and shred chicken using a knife and fork.

2

Bring 4 cups water to a boil; add noodles and cook until tender, about 5 minutes. Add chicken, peas and carrots, and egg yolks; cook over high heat, stirring constantly, until soup is heated through, about 5 minutes. Add scallions and soy sauce; cook for 2 minutes more.

3

Transfer soup to bowls and serve with kimchi on the side.

NUTRITION FACTS:

726 calories; protein 60.5g; carbohydrates 67.7g; fat 23.7g;

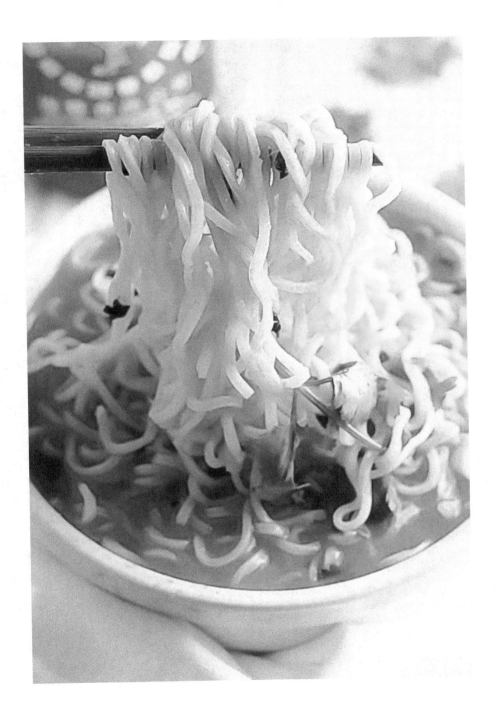

CHAPTER 3: **SALAD RECIPES**

Easy Smoky Kale Salad

Prep:

30 mins

Total:

30 mins

Servings:

8

Yield:

8 servings

INGREDIENTS:

Salad:

⅔ cup grated Gouda cheese

⅔ cup pitted and chopped Kalamata olives

⅔ cup thinly-sliced sun-dried tomatoes

1 ⅓ pounds kale, stems removed and leaves chopped

2 ⅓ cups frozen baby lima beans, thawed

Dressing:

1 tablespoon ground chipotle chile pepper

2 ⅔ teaspoons balsamic vinegar

2 teaspoons ground black pepper

1 ¾ teaspoons kosher salt

1 ⅓ cups olive oil

½ cup lemon juice

2 ⅔ tablespoons smoked paprika

2 ½ tablespoons honey

DIRECTIONS:

1

Mix kale, lima beans, Gouda cheese, Kalamata olives, and sun-dried tomatoes together in a bowl.

2

Whisk olive oil, lemon juice, paprika, honey, chipotle pepper, balsamic vinegar, black pepper, and kosher salt together in a bowl until dressing is smooth; pour over kale mixture and toss to coat.

NUTRITION FACTS:

511 calories; protein 8.4g; carbohydrates 33.1g; fat 40.8g;

Black Bean and Couscous Salad

Prep:

30 mins

Additional:

5 mins

Total:

35 mins

Servings:

8

Yield:

8 to 10 servings

INGREDIENTS:

8 green onions, chopped

1 red bell pepper, seeded and chopped

¼ cup chopped fresh cilantro

1 cup frozen corn kernels, thawed

2 (15 ounce) cans black beans, drained

salt and pepper to taste

1 cup uncooked couscous

1 ¼ cups chicken broth

3 tablespoons extra virgin olive oil

2 tablespoons fresh lime juice

1 teaspoon red wine vinegar

½ teaspoon ground cumin

DIRECTIONS:

1

Bring chicken broth to a boil in a 2 quart or larger sauce pan and stir in the couscous. Cover the pot and remove from heat. Let stand for 5 minutes.

2

In a large bowl, whisk together the olive oil, lime juice, vinegar and cumin. Add green onions, red pepper, cilantro, corn and beans and toss to coat.

3

Fluff the couscous well, breaking up any chunks. Add to the bowl with the vegetables and mix well. Season with salt and pepper to taste and serve at once or refrigerate until ready to serve.

NUTRITION FACTS:

253 calories; protein 10.3g; carbohydrates 41.1g; fat 5.8g;

Warm Green Bean and Potato Salad with Goat Cheese

Prep:

15 mins

Cook:

15 mins

Total:

30 mins

Servings:

8

Yield:

8 servings

INGREDIENTS:

4 cloves minced garlic

½ cup reduced-fat balsamic vinaigrette dressing

1 cup jarred roasted red peppers, drained and chopped

¼ cup chopped fresh basil

1 (8 ounce) package goat cheese, crumbled

2 pounds red potatoes, cut into bite-size pieces

1 serving olive oil cooking spray

½ pound frozen French-style green beans, thawed

1 cup chopped red onion

DIRECTIONS:

1

Place the potatoes into a large pot and cover with salted water. Bring to a boil over high heat, then reduce heat to medium-low, cover, and simmer until tender, 8 to 10 minutes. Drain and allow to steam dry for a minute or two. Place potatoes in a large bowl.

2

Heat a large skillet over medium-high heat; grease with cooking spray. Cook and stir the green beans and onion until tender, about 5 minutes. Stir in the garlic; cook and stir until garlic is fragrant, about 1 minute more.

3

Transfer the green bean mixture into the large bowl with the potatoes. Add the balsamic vinaigrette, roasted red peppers, and basil; toss lightly. Stir in the goat cheese.

NUTRITION FACTS:

252 calories; protein 9.2g; carbohydrates 28.6g; fat 9.6g;

Fennel and Avocado Salad

Prep:

10 mins

Total:

10 mins

Servings:

4

Yield:

4 servings

INGREDIENTS:

2 tablespoons extra-virgin olive oil, or to taste

1 teaspoon ground nutmeg

salt to taste

3 bulbs fennel, thinly sliced

1 avocado - peeled, pitted, and cubed

DIRECTIONS:

1

Mix fennel and avocado together in a bowl. Stir in oil, nutmeg, and salt; mix until well combined.

NUTRITION FACTS:

119 calories; protein 2.2g; carbohydrates 13.2g; fat 7.4g;

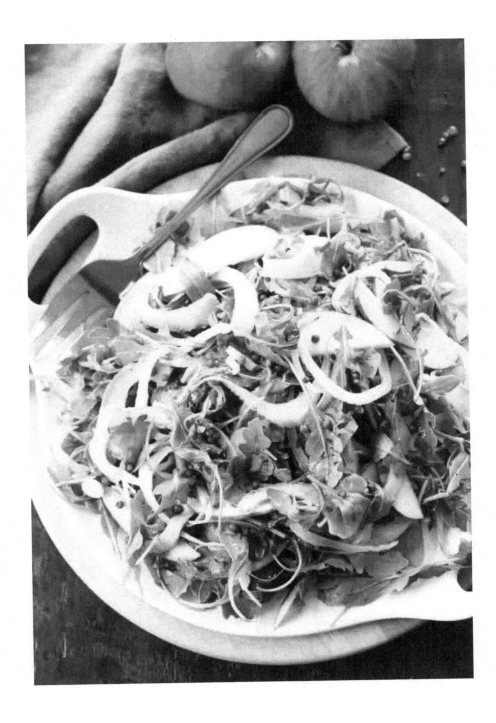

CHAPTER 4: **LUNCH & DINNER RECIPES**

Mushroom Curry with Galangal

Prep:

10 mins

Cook:

20 mins

Total:

30 mins

Servings:

4

Yield:

4 servings

INGREDIENTS:

⅓ pound sliced fresh mushrooms

5 Thai chile peppers, chopped

¼ cup fresh lime juice

1 tablespoon fish sauce

2 cups coconut milk

1 (2 inch) piece galangal, peeled and sliced

3 kaffir lime leaves, torn

2 teaspoons salt

DIRECTIONS:

1

Put the coconut milk and galangal in a pot and bring to a boil. Add the kaffir lime leaves and salt; simmer for 10 minutes. Add the mushrooms and cook until soft, 5 to 7 minutes. Remove from heat. Stir the lime juice and fish sauce into the mixture; pour into a bowl and top with the Thai chilies to serve.

NUTRITION FACTS:

261 calories; protein 4.9g; carbohydrates 11.8g; fat 24.4g;

Green Bean and Portobello Mushroom Casserole

Prep:

15 mins

Cook:

35 mins

Total:

50 mins

Servings:

10

Yield:

10 servings

INGREDIENTS:

½ cup slivered almonds

1 (10.75 ounce) can condensed cream of mushroom soup with roasted garlic

¾ teaspoon seasoned salt with no MSG

⅓ teaspoon white pepper

2 (15.5 ounce) cans French cut green beans, drained

1 cup shredded Cheddar cheese

4 slices bacon

¼ cup olive oil

1 pound baby portobello mushrooms, sliced

½ medium onion, chopped

3 cloves garlic, finely chopped

DIRECTIONS:

1

Preheat the oven to 375 degrees F (190 degrees C).

2

Place bacon in a large skillet over medium-high heat, and fry until crisp. Remove from the skillet to drain on paper towels. Pour olive oil into the skillet, and reduce heat to medium. When oil is hot, add mushrooms and onion; cook, stirring frequently until the onions start to become translucent. Add garlic, and fry for a couple of minutes, just until fragrant. Stir in the mushroom soup and almonds, and bring to a boil. Season with seasoned salt and white pepper, and crumble in the bacon. Gently stir in the green beans, then transfer the mixture to a casserole dish.

3

Bake uncovered for 30 minutes in the preheated oven. Remove from the oven, and sprinkle Cheddar cheese over the top. Return to the oven for 5 minutes, or until cheese is melted. Let stand 5 minutes before serving.

NUTRITION FACTS:

244 calories; protein 8.5g; carbohydrates 10.3g; fat 19.3g;

Beet Salad on a Stick

Prep:

15 mins

Total:

15 mins

Servings:

8

Yield:

8 servings

INGREDIENTS:

8 (2 ounce) roasted beet wedges

24 fresh spinach leaves

3 tablespoons honey

3 tablespoons chopped walnuts

8 ounces chilled goat cheese, rolled into 8 balls

8 bamboo toothpicks

DIRECTIONS:

1

Pour walnuts into a shallow bowl. Roll goat cheese balls in walnuts to coat completely.

2

Thread 1 coated goat cheese ball onto a toothpick; add beet wedge and 4 baby spinach leaves to the toothpick. Repeat with remaining toothpicks, goat cheese, beets, and spinach. Drizzle each skewer with honey.

NUTRITION FACTS:

177 calories; protein 8.4g; carbohydrates 14.3g; fat 10.5g;

Creamy Asparagus Pasta

Prep:

5 mins

Cook:

25 mins

Total:

30 mins

Servings:

8

Yield:

8 servings

INGREDIENTS:

1 pint light cream

1 pound linguine pasta

1 lemon, juiced

1 pound fresh asparagus, trimmed and cut into 2 inch pieces

2 tablespoons butter

1 clove garlic, minced

DIRECTIONS:

1

Bring a pot of water to a boil. Boil asparagus for 3 to 4 minutes; drain.

2

In a large saucepan melt butter over medium heat. Saute garlic and asparagus for 3 to 4 minutes. Stir in the cream and simmer for 10 minutes.

3

Meanwhile, bring a large pot of water to a boil. Add linguine and cook for 8 to 10 minutes or until al dente; drain and transfer to a serving dish.

4

Stir lemon juice into asparagus mixture; pour mixture over pasta.

NUTRITION FACTS:

247 calories; protein 8.3g; carbohydrates 44g; fat 4.7g;

Veggie and Goat Cheese Quinoa Burgers

Prep:

20 mins

Cook:

12 mins

Additional:

30 mins

Total:

1 hr 2 mins

Servings:

4

Yield:

4 burgers

INGREDIENTS:

2 tablespoons vegetable oil

4 slices Perfectly Crafted Multigrain Bread, toasted

4 leaves Fresh basil

⅓ cup Diced tomato

¼ cup Sliced red onion

1 cup cooked quinoa

1 cup canned pumpkin

¾ cup fresh basil, chopped

1 medium beet, peeled and shredded

½ cup quick-cooking oats

½ cup soft, spreadable goat cheese, divided

2 cloves garlic, minced

½ teaspoon salt

½ teaspoon ground ginger

DIRECTIONS:

1

In a large bowl, combine quinoa, pumpkin, 3/4 cup basil, beet, oats, 1/4 cup goat cheese, garlic, salt, and ginger. Mix until well combined. Cover and chill for 30 minutes or until easy to work with.

2

In a very large skillet, heat oil over medium heat. Meanwhile, divide the mixture into 4 portions and press each portion into a 4-inch patty.

3

Cook patties in hot oil over medium heat for 12 to 15 minutes or until firm and lightly browned, turning once halfway through cooking.

4

Spread remaining 1/4 cup goat cheese over toasted bread slices. Top with quinoa burgers. If desired, garnish with additional fresh basil, diced tomato, and/or sliced red onion.

NUTRITION FACTS:

304 calories; protein 8.6g; carbohydrates 45.7g; fat 10.9g;

Brussels Sprouts Stir Fry

Prep:

20 mins

Cook:

15 mins

Total:

35 mins

Servings:

8

Yield:

8 servings

INGREDIENTS:

1 red pepper, seeded and cut into 1/2-inch cubes

¼ cup chicken broth

ground black pepper, to taste

2 tablespoons chopped green onions

1 tablespoon vegetable oil

1 onion, chopped

1 large potato, peeled and cubed

1 bay leaf

1 pound Brussels sprouts, trimmed and halved lengthwise

DIRECTIONS:

1

Heat the vegetable oil in a skillet over medium heat. Stir in the onion, potato, and bay leaf. Cook and stir until the onion is transparent, about 5 minutes. Add the Brussels sprouts, red pepper, and chicken broth. Cover and cook until vegetables are tender, about 10 minutes. Remove the bay leaf. Toss with black pepper, to taste. Garnish with green onions, and serve immediately.

NUTRITION FACTS:

86 calories; protein 3.2g; carbohydrates 15.5g; fat 2g;

Couscous Caprese

Prep:

10 mins

Cook:

20 mins

Additional:

5 mins

Total:

35 mins

Servings:

4

Yield:

4 servings

INGREDIENTS:

16 leaves fresh basil

8 ounces fresh mozzarella cheese, diced

1 cup boiling water

1 cup couscous

4 tomatoes

¼ cup balsamic vinegar, or to taste

DIRECTIONS:

1

Preheat oven to 350 degrees F (175 degrees C). Lightly grease a baking dish.

2

Pour boiling water over couscous in a bowl. Cover bowl with plastic wrap. Let couscous soak until the water is completely absorbed, about 5 minutes.

3

Slice the tops from tomatoes and take a very small slice of the bottoms so they will be stable upright. Use a spoon to remove and discard the tomato innards. Put tomatoes in the prepared baking dish.

4

Bake tomatoes in the preheated oven until lightly charred at the edges, about 20 minutes.

5

Line the inner walls of each tomato with 4 basil leaves.

6

Toss mozzarella cheese with the couscous; stuff into tomatoes. Drizzle balsamic vinegar over the top of the stuffed tomatoes.

NUTRITION FACTS:

292 calories; protein 18.8g; carbohydrates 32.6g; fat 9.4g;

Fried Rice Bowl

Prep:

30 mins

Cook:

30 mins

Total:

1 hr

Servings:

6

Yield:

6 servings

INGREDIENTS:

3 tablespoons vegetable oil, or as needed

1 cup cubed carrots

1 cup chopped yellow onion

4 tablespoons minced fresh ginger root

4 tablespoons minced garlic

½ cup thinly sliced green onions

1 cup frozen peas

3 tablespoons tamari

2 tablespoons sesame oil

fresh ground black pepper

6 sticks dried bean curd

1 tablespoon shredded black fungus

7 dried black mushrooms

boiling water

3 ¼ cups water

2 cups basmati rice

1 tablespoon butter or oil

4 eggs, beaten

DIRECTIONS:

1

Place the dried bean curd in a bowl, and cover with boiling water. In a smaller bowl, place the shredded black fungus and dried black mushrooms, and cover with boiling water. Allow the bean curd, black fungus, and dried black mushrooms to soak until rehydrated, about 20 minutes.

2

Place 3 1/4 cups of water with rice in a saucepan. Bring to a boil over high heat, and let it boil hard for one minute. Cover with a lid, and turn heat to low. Cook on low for 5 minutes, then remove from heat (without lifting the lid). Let sit, covered, while you prepare the rest of the meal, or about 20 minutes. Do not at any time lift the lid.

3

In a non-stick skillet, melt butter over medium-high heat. Scramble eggs to the dry instead of the creamy point. Dump them into a bowl, and continue to chop them into bits with the edge of a wooden spoon. You don't have to pulverize them, go for pieces about the size of your thumbnail.

4

In one bowl, combine carrot, onion, garlic, and ginger. In another bowl, green onions and frozen peas. Now drain all the water off the bean curd, fungus and mushrooms. The bean curd might need some tough bits removed, and the remainder cut into quarter-inch rings. The mushrooms only need slicing and the fungus is pre-sliced so no worries there. Combine bean curd and mushrooms in a third bowl.

5

Heat wok over high heat; let the metal get smoking hot, about one minute. Add three tablespoons of vegetable oil. Wait about 30 seconds, and tip in the bowl of carrot, onion, garlic, and ginger. Cook, stirring frequently. The garlic's going to brown first because it has the highest sugar content, so keep an eye on it, and turn the flame down if necessary. Tip in the bean curd, shredded fungus, and mushrooms, and cook and stir for one minute. Now look to see that your flame is set to maximum, and tip in the spring onion and the frozen peas. You don't need to cook them, just threaten them. Keep them moving, and mix in the rice. Stir in the eggs, and then season with generous, generous amounts of tamari and sesame oil, and a few twists of fresh black pepper.

NUTRITION FACTS:

539 calories; protein 19.9g; carbohydrates 71.7g; fat 19.8g;

Vegetarian Bolognese with Soy Chorizo

Prep:

10 mins

Cook:

15 mins

Total:

25 mins

Servings:

8

Yield:

8 servings

INGREDIENTS:

12 ounces soy chorizo

1 teaspoon dried oregano

½ teaspoon cayenne pepper

½ teaspoon paprika

2 teaspoons chopped fresh basil

½ teaspoon freshly ground black pepper

fine sea salt to taste

3 cups water

1 (16 ounce) package thin spaghetti

1 tablespoon olive oil

18 ounces marinara sauce

1 (14.5 ounce) can diced tomatoes

DIRECTIONS:

1

Bring about 3 cups lightly salted water to a boil in a medium-sized pot. Add pasta and cook, stirring occasionally, until tender yet firm to the bite, about 11 minutes.

2

Meanwhile, heat olive oil over medium heat in a large skillet. Add marinara sauce and diced tomatoes and stir. Add soy chorizo and mix until texture is even, 3 to 5 minutes. Add oregano, cayenne pepper, and paprika; reduce heat and simmer until pasta has finished cooking, about 8 minutes more. Add basil.

3

Drain cooked pasta; top with sauce. Season with black pepper and salt.

NUTRITION FACTS:

386 calories; protein 15.5g; carbohydrates 57.9g; fat 10.3g;

Fajita Vegetable Stir-Fry

Prep:

10 mins

Cook:

10 mins

Total:

20 mins

Servings:

4

Yield:

4 servings

INGREDIENTS:

2 tablespoons Country Spread

2 medium red or yellow bell peppers, sliced

1 medium sweet onion, cut into thin wedges

1 clove garlic, finely chopped

½ teaspoon ground cumin

¼ teaspoon chili powder

1 tablespoon lime juice

1 tablespoon chopped fresh cilantro

DIRECTIONS:

1

Melt Country Spread in 12-inch nonstick skillet over medium-high heat and cook red peppers and onion until tender and golden, about 8 minutes. Stir in garlic, cumin and chili powder and cook, stirring frequently, 2 minutes. Remove from heat, stir in lime juice and cilantro.

NUTRITION FACTS:

33 calories; protein 1g; carbohydrates 6.9g; fat 0.3g;

Bean & pecan sandwiches

Prep:

20 mins

Cook:

22 mins

Additional:

3 mins

Total:

45 mins

Servings:

8

Yield:

8 servings

INGREDIENTS:

1 medium onion, thinly sliced

2 medium tomatoes, cut into 1/4 inch slices

4 slices Cheddar cheese

4 slices bacon

4 English muffins, split

1 (16 ounce) can maple cured baked beans

DIRECTIONS:

1

Preheat oven to 350 degrees F (175 degrees C).

2

Arrange the English muffin halves on a baking sheet. Place an equal amount of baked beans on each muffin half. Layer beans with onion, tomato, cheese, and bacon.

3

Bake 20 minutes in the preheated oven. Set oven to broil, and continue cooking 1 to 2 minutes, until bacon is crisp. Watch constantly during broiling to make sure bacon does not burn. Serve immediately.

NUTRITION FACTS:

225 calories; protein 10.9g; carbohydrates 28.5g; fat 7.4g;

Cuban Inspired Millet

Prep:

20 mins

Cook:

35 mins

Total:

55 mins

Servings:

8

Yield:

8 servings

INGREDIENTS:

1 green bell pepper, chopped

1 cup millet

2 cups vegetable broth

salt and ground black pepper to taste

1 carrot, chopped

2 cloves garlic, crushed

1 tablespoon olive oil

1 onion, chopped

¼ cup chopped fresh cilantro, or more to taste

DIRECTIONS:

1

Blend carrot and garlic in a food processor until finely chopped.

2

Heat olive oil in a pot over medium heat; cook and stir carrot mixture, onion, and green bell pepper until softened, about 10 minutes. Add millet; stir until fragrant and toasted, about 3 minutes.

3

Pour vegetable broth into millet mixture; season with salt and black pepper. Reduce heat and simmer until all the broth is absorbed and millet is tender, about 20 minutes. Stir in cilantro.

NUTRITION FACTS:

130 calories; protein 3.4g; carbohydrates 22.5g; fat 2.9g;

Buckwheat Granola

Prep:

10 mins

Cook:

40 mins

Additional:

1 hr

Total:

1 hr 50 mins

Servings:

10

Yield:

10 servings

INGREDIENTS:

¼ cup honey

1 vanilla bean, split and scraped

½ cup almonds, chopped

½ cup sweetened flaked coconut

½ cup raisins

2 cups rolled oats

¾ cup buckwheat groats, chopped

¾ cup sunflower seeds

1 pinch salt

3 tablespoons coconut oil

DIRECTIONS:

1

Preheat oven to 300 degrees F (150 degrees C). Line a baking sheet with parchment paper.

2

Mix oats, buckwheat, sunflower seeds, and salt in a large bowl.

3

Melt coconut oil in a small saucepan over medium heat; stir in honey and seeds from vanilla bean until mixed. Pour over oat mixture and toss to coat. Spread oat mixture evenly over prepared baking sheet.

4

Bake in the preheated oven, stirring every 10 minutes, until granola is lightly brown, 35 to 40 minutes. Stir almonds into granola and continue baking until golden grown, about 5 to 10 minutes more. Allow granola to cool completely, then stir in coconut and raisins. Store in an airtight container.

NUTRITION FACTS:

304 calories; protein 7.5g; carbohydrates 40g; fat 14.6g

Baked Asparagus and Mushroom Pasta

Prep:

20 mins

Cook:

40 mins

Total:

1 hr

Servings:

6

Yield:

1 7x11-inch casserole

INGREDIENTS:

¼ teaspoon crushed red pepper flakes

1 pinch salt and ground black pepper to taste

2 tablespoons unsalted butter

2 tablespoons all-purpose flour

2 cups 1% milk

⅔ cup grated Parmigiano-Reggiano cheese, divided

¼ cup shredded provolone cheese

½ (16 ounce) package gemelli pasta

2 tablespoons herb-infused extra-virgin olive oil

½ medium onion, chopped

1 pound fresh asparagus, cut into 1-inch pieces

1 (8 ounce) package sliced mushrooms

2 cups cherry tomatoes, halved

2 cloves garlic, minced

⅓ cup Italian-seasoned bread crumbs

DIRECTIONS:

1

Preheat the oven to 350 degrees F (175 degrees C). Grease a 7x11-inch baking dish.

2

Bring a large pot of lightly salted water to a boil; cook gemelli at a boil until flexible but still firm to the bite, about 6 minutes.

3

Meanwhile, heat oil in a large skillet over medium heat until shimmering. Add onion and stir for 2 minutes. Add asparagus and mushrooms and continue to cook, stirring occasionally, until mushrooms begin to soften and asparagus is bright green, about 4 minutes.

4

Add tomatoes, garlic, red pepper flakes, salt, and pepper. Continue cooking for about 4 minutes, stirring occasionally.

5

Pour the vegetable mixture into a large mixing bowl. Drain pasta and stir into the bowl.

6

Melt butter in the same skillet. Add flour and cook, stirring constantly, until the mixture bubbles, about 4 minutes. Pour in milk, stirring briskly to avoid lumps. Continue to stir until sauce thickens and bubbles again, about 4 minutes. Remove from heat and stir in 1/3 cup Parmigiano-Reggiano and provolone cheese until melted.

7

Pour the cheese sauce over the pasta and vegetables and stir to combine. Pour into the prepared baking dish. Taste and adjust seasonings. Toss remaining Parmigiano-Reggiano with bread crumbs and sprinkle over the casserole.

8

Bake in the preheated oven until bubbly and lightly browned, 20 to 25 minutes.

NUTRITION FACTS:

356 calories; protein 15.9g; carbohydrates 46.1g; fat 13.3g;

Holiday Oyster Stuffing

Prep:

15 mins

Cook:

1 hr

Total:

1 hr 15 mins

Servings:

10

Yield:

10 servings

INGREDIENTS:

salt and ground black pepper to taste

1 ½ cups turkey broth

¼ cup margarine

1 (6 ounce) package corn bread stuffing mix

1 pound bulk pork sausage

1 pound ground beef (Optional)

1 small onion, chopped

1 egg, beaten

1 pint shucked oysters, drained, or more if desired

1 turkey giblets, cooked and chopped

1 teaspoon poultry seasoning

DIRECTIONS:

1

Preheat oven to 350 degrees F (175 degrees C). Grease a 9x9-inch baking dish.

2

Bring the turkey broth to a boil in a saucepan over medium heat, and melt the margarine in the broth. Stir in the stuffing mix until thoroughly combined. Transfer the stuffing to a large bowl. Stir in pork sausage, ground beef, onion, and egg until the mixture is well combined, and lightly mix in the oysters, turkey giblets, poultry seasoning, salt, and black pepper. Transfer the oyster stuffing to the prepared baking dish, and cover dish with foil.

3

Bake in the preheated oven until the sausage and ground beef are cooked through and the stuffing is crisp and lightly browned, about 1 hour.

NUTRITION FACTS:

391 calories; protein 26.9g; carbohydrates 17.1g; fat 23.2g;

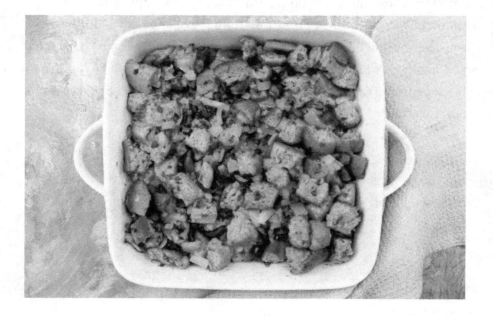

CHAPTER 5: **SNACK E SIDES RECIPES**

Mushroom Curry with Galangal

Prep:

10 mins

Cook:

20 mins

Total:

30 mins

Servings:

4

Yield:

4 servings

INGREDIENTS:

⅓ pound sliced fresh mushrooms

5 Thai chile peppers, chopped

¼ cup fresh lime juice

2 cups coconut milk

1 (2 inch) piece galangal, peeled and sliced

3 kaffir lime leaves, torn

2 teaspoons salt

1 tablespoon fish sauce

DIRECTIONS:

1

Put the coconut milk and galangal in a pot and bring to a boil. Add the kaffir lime leaves and salt; simmer for 10 minutes. Add the mushrooms and cook until soft, 5 to 7 minutes. Remove from heat. Stir the lime juice and fish sauce into the mixture; pour into a bowl and top with the Thai chilies to serve.

NUTRITION FACTS:

261 calories; protein 4.9g; carbohydrates 11.8g; fat 24.4g;

Roasted Garlic Cauliflower Mash

Prep:

10 mins

Cook:

40 mins

Total:

50 mins

Servings:

6

Yield:

6 servings

INGREDIENTS:

1 teaspoon kosher salt

1 teaspoon dried parsley

¼ teaspoon ground black pepper

6 cloves garlic, crushed

3 tablespoons olive oil

1 large head cauliflower, coarsely chopped

DIRECTIONS:

1

Preheat oven to 350 degrees F (175 degrees C).

2

Place garlic in a casserole dish and drizzle with olive oil.

3

Roast garlic in the preheated oven until tender and fragrant, about 15 minutes.

4

Place a steamer insert into a saucepan and fill with water to just below the bottom of the steamer. Bring water to a boil. Add cauliflower, cover, and steam until tender, about 10 minutes.

5

Mash cauliflower and roasted garlic with olive oil together in a bowl. Stir salt, parsley, and pepper into mashed cauliflower until completely incorporated. Spread cauliflower mixture into casserole dish.

6

Bake mashed cauliflower in the preheated oven until hot and flavors blend, about 15 minutes.

NUTRITION FACTS:

100 calories; protein 3g; carbohydrates 8.5g; fat 6.9g;

Vegan Potato Soy Chorizo Tacos

Prep:

10 mins

Cook:

43 mins

Total:

53 mins

Servings:

4

Yield:

4 servings

INGREDIENTS:

2 tablespoons vegetable oil, divided

12 ounces soy chorizo, crumbled

12 (6 inch) corn tortillas

2 pounds Yukon Gold potatoes, peeled

salt and ground black pepper to taste

DIRECTIONS:

1

Place potatoes in a large pot and cover with salted water; bring to a boil. Cook, covered, until potatoes are easily pierced with a knife, about 30 minutes. Drain, reserving 1 cup cooking water.

2

Transfer boiled potatoes to a bowl and season with salt and pepper. Mash with a potato masher, adding reserved cooking water to reach desired consistency.

3

Heat 1 tablespoon oil in a large skillet. Cook soy chorizo for 5 minutes. Add mashed potatoes and mix well.

4

Heat tortillas on a hot griddle over medium heat to soften them. Fill them with equal amounts of potato-chorizo mixture. Fold them in half and brush the outside of the tortillas with the remaining 1 tablespoon oil. Place tacos on the hot griddle and cook, turning once, until crisp, 3 to 5 minutes.

NUTRITION FACTS:

597 calories; protein 22.2g; carbohydrates 85.2g; fat 21.2g;

Garlic Pepper Seitan

Prep:

10 mins

Cook:

45 mins

Total:

55 mins

Servings:

4

Yield:

4 servings

INGREDIENTS:

2 (8 ounce) packages chicken style seitan

½ teaspoon ground black pepper

salt to taste

1 tablespoon cornstarch

2 tablespoons cold water ¼ cup olive oil

½ cup chopped onion

5 cloves garlic, finely minced

¼ cup chopped green bell pepper

DIRECTIONS:

1

Heat olive oil in a skillet over medium-low heat. Add onions and garlic, and cook, stirring until lightly browned. Increase the heat to medium, and add the green pepper and seitan to the pan, stirring to coat the seitan evenly. Season with salt and pepper. Reduce heat to low, cover, and simmer for 35 minutes in order for the seitan to absorb the flavors. Dissolve cornstarch in cold water, and stir into the skillet. Cook, stirring until thickened, and serve immediately.

NUTRITION FACTS:

301 calories; protein 26.3g; carbohydrates 15.3g; fat 15.6g;

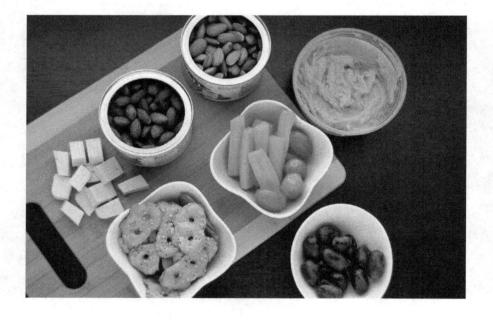

CHAPTER 6: **DESSERT**

Southern Summer Squash Pudding

Prep:

15 mins

Cook:

1 hr 5 mins

Additional:

30 mins

Total:

1 hr 50 mins

Servings:

24

Yield:

24 servings

INGREDIENTS:

1 egg, beaten

2 tablespoons butter, melted

2 teaspoons lemon extract

1 cup self-rising flour

3 ¼ cups peeled, seeded, and diced yellow squash

1 ½ cups white sugar

½ cup milk

DIRECTIONS:

1

Place a steamer insert into a saucepan and fill with water to just below the bottom of the steamer. Bring water to a boil. Add squash, cover, and steam until tender, 2 to 6 minutes. Transfer squash to a bowl and mash with a fork or potato masher until smooth.

2

Preheat oven to 350 degrees F (175 degrees C). Generously grease a 9x13-inch baking dish.

3

Combine sugar, milk, egg, butter, and lemon extract in a large bowl. Gradually sift flour into milk mixture. Fold mashed squash into milk mixture until batter is smooth. Pour batter into prepared baking dish.

4

Bake in the preheated oven until air bubbles form on the surface and pudding is golden brown, about 1 hour. Chill in the refrigerator until firm; cut into bars.

NUTRITION FACTS:

85 calories; protein 1.1g; carbohydrates 17.3g; fat 1.4g;

Vanilla Pudding

Servings:

5

Yield:

5 to 6 servings

INGREDIENTS:

¼ teaspoon salt

2 ½ cups milk

1 ½ teaspoons vanilla extract

⅓ cup white sugar

3 tablespoons cornstarch

DIRECTIONS:

1

In a saucepan, combine the sugar, corn starch and salt. Add milk and cook over medium heat, stirring constantly until mixture thickens. Add vanilla and continue to cook for 2 to 3 minutes.

2

Pour into individual molds rinsed with cold water; chill until firm and unmold.

NUTRITION FACTS:

135 calories; protein 4g; carbohydrates 23.6g; fat 2.4g;

White Chocolate Fudge with Pecans

Prep:

14 mins

Cook:

1 min

Additional:

1 hr

Total:

1 hr 15 mins

Servings:

16

Yield:

16 servings

INGREDIENTS:

½ teaspoon vanilla extract

1 (12 ounce) package white chocolate chips

¾ cup chopped pecans (Optional)

1 (8 ounce) package cream cheese, softened

4 cups confectioners' sugar

DIRECTIONS:

1

Grease an 8x8-inch baking dish with butter.

2

Beat cream cheese in a bowl with an electric mixer until light and fluffy. Gradually beat in confectioners' sugar and vanilla extract until smooth.

3

Melt chocolate in a microwave-safe bowl in 30-second intervals, stirring after each melting, for 1 to 3 minutes (depending on your microwave). Beat chocolate into cream cheese mixture until smooth. Stir in pecans. Pour chocolate mixture into prepared baking dish. Chill until set.

NUTRITION FACTS:

326 calories; protein 3g; carbohydrates 44.3g; fat 16.1g;

Chocolate Peanut Butter Cup Cookies

Prep:

15 mins

Cook:

10 mins

Additional:

45 mins

Total:

1 hr 10 mins

Servings:

36

Yield:

3 dozen

INGREDIENTS:

⅓ cup cocoa powder

1 teaspoon baking soda

1 cup semisweet chocolate chips

1 cup peanut butter chips

10 chocolate covered peanut butter cups, cut into eighths

1 cup butter, softened

¾ cup creamy peanut butter

¾ cup white sugar

¾ cup packed brown sugar

2 eggs

1 teaspoon vanilla extract

2 ⅓ cups all-purpose flour

DIRECTIONS:

1

Preheat oven to 350 degrees F (175 degrees C).

2

In a large bowl, cream together the butter, peanut butter, white sugar, and brown sugar until smooth. Beat in the eggs one at a time, then stir in the vanilla. Combine the flour, cocoa, and baking soda; stir into the peanut butter mixture. Mix in the chocolate chips, peanut butter chips, and peanut butter cups. Drop by tablespoonfuls onto ungreased cookie sheets.

3

Bake for 8 to 10 minutes in the preheated oven. Let cool for 1 or 2 minutes on sheet before removing, or they will fall apart.

NUTRITION FACTS:

230 calories; protein 4.8g; carbohydrates 25.2g; fat 13g;

Carrot Cupcakes with White Chocolate Cream Cheese Icing

Prep:

30 mins

Cook:

25 mins

Additional:

1 hr

Total:

1 hr 55 mins

Servings:

12

Yield:

12 muffin

INGREDIENTS:

Cream Cheese Icing:

2 ounces white chocolate

1 (8 ounce) package cream cheese, softened

½ cup unsalted butter, softened

1 teaspoon vanilla extract

½ teaspoon orange extract

4 cups confectioners' sugar

2 tablespoons heavy cream

Carrot Cake:

2 eggs, lightly beaten

1 ⅛ cups white sugar

⅓ cup brown sugar

½ teaspoon salt

1 ½ teaspoons ground cinnamon

½ teaspoon ground nutmeg

¼ teaspoon ground ginger

1 cup chopped walnuts

½ cup vegetable oil

1 teaspoon vanilla extract

2 cups shredded carrots

½ cup crushed pineapple

1 ½ cups all-purpose flour

1 ¼ teaspoons baking soda

DIRECTIONS:

1

Preheat oven to 350 degrees F (175 degrees C). Lightly grease 12 muffin cups.

2

In small saucepan, melt white chocolate over low heat. Stir until smooth, and allow to cool to room temperature.

3

In a bowl, beat together the cream cheese and butter until smooth. Mix in white chocolate, 1 teaspoon vanilla, and orange extract. Gradually beat in the confectioners' sugar until the mixture is fluffy. Mix in heavy cream.

4

Beat together the eggs, white sugar, and brown sugar in a bowl, and mix in the oil and vanilla. Fold in carrots and pineapple. In a separate bowl, mix the flour, baking soda, salt, cinnamon, nutmeg, and ginger. Mix flour mixture into the carrot mixture until evenly moist. Fold in 1/2 cup walnuts. Transfer to the prepared muffin cups.

5

Bake 25 minutes in the preheated oven, or until a toothpick inserted in the center of a muffin comes out clean. Cool completely on wire racks before topping with the icing and sprinkling with remaining walnuts.

NUTRITION FACTS:

639 calories; protein 6g; carbohydrates 84.7g; fat 32.2g;

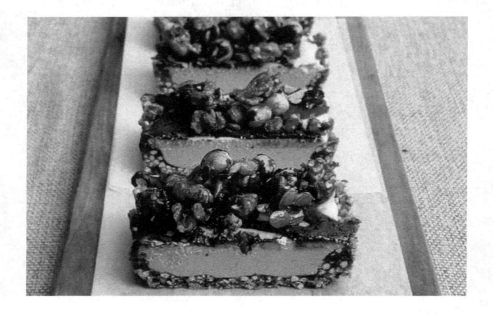

CHAPTER 7: **HOMEMADE SAUCE E CONDIMENTS RECIPES**

Cashew Cheese Sauce

Prep:

10 mins

Cook:

10 mins

Additional:

10 mins

Total:

30 mins

Servings:

5

Yield:

5 servings

INGREDIENTS:

2 tablespoons cornstarch

2 tablespoons classic deli mustard

ground black pepper to taste

1 cup raw cashews

2 cups water, or more as needed

4 tablespoons nutritional yeast flakes

DIRECTIONS:

1

Rinse cashews under warm water. Place in a bowl and cover with hot water. Let soak for 10 minutes.

2

Combine 2 cups water, nutritional yeast, cornstarch, and mustard in a blender or food processor. Blend on high for 1 minute. Add soaked cashews and blend on high until smooth, 1 1/2 minutes or longer. Transfer to a medium saucepan.

3

Cook over low heat, whisking constantly, until sauce thickens, 5 to 7 minutes. Add more water if needed to reach desired consistency. Season with black pepper.

NUTRITION FACTS:

196 calories; protein 7.4g; carbohydrates 15.3g; fat 13g;

Maple Salad Dressing

Prep:

10 mins

Total:

10 mins

Servings:

14

Yield:

1 3/4 cup

INGREDIENTS:

1 teaspoon dry mustard

1 teaspoon salt

½ teaspoon dried basil

¼ teaspoon ground black pepper

1 cup extra-virgin olive oil

½ cup pure maple syrup

¼ cup balsamic vinegar

1 tablespoon fresh lemon juice

1 clove garlic, minced

DIRECTIONS:

1

Blend maple syrup, balsamic vinegar, lemon juice, garlic, dry mustard, salt, basil, and black pepper in a blender until smooth; stream olive oil into the mixture while blending and continue blending until dressing is thick and creamy.

NUTRITION FACTS:

178 calories; protein 0.1g; carbohydrates 8.5g; fat 16.1g;

Soy Milk Vegan Mayo

Prep:

10 mins

Total:

10 mins

Servings:

24

Yield:

3 cups

INGREDIENTS:

1 teaspoon garlic powder

1 teaspoon onion powder

½ teaspoon dried dill weed, crushed

½ teaspoon ground turmeric

1 pinch cayenne pepper

2 cups olive oil

1 cup soy milk

2 tablespoons cider vinegar

4 teaspoons dry mustard

1 teaspoon sea salt

1 pinch curry powder

DIRECTIONS:

1

Combine olive oil, soy milk, vinegar, mustard, salt, garlic powder, onion powder, dill, turmeric, cayenne, and curry in a food processor; blend until thick. Store in the refrigerator.

NUTRITION FACTS:

169 calories; protein 0.5g; carbohydrates 1g; fat 18.4g;

Tofu Mayonnaise

Prep:

10 mins

Total:

10 mins

Servings:

16

Yield:

2 cups

INGREDIENTS:

1 teaspoon dry mustard

1 teaspoon salt

½ teaspoon pepper

¼ cup peanut oil

1 (12 ounce) package tofu, drained and cut into cubes

½ teaspoon sesame oil

2 tablespoons apple cider vinegar

DIRECTIONS:

1

Place the tofu, sesame oil, cider vinegar, mustard, salt and pepper into the container of a blender. Blend until smooth. Drizzle the peanut oil in a thin stream while blending until thick and pale. Use promptly.

NUTRITION FACTS:

49 calories; protein 1.8g; carbohydrates 0.5g; fat 4.6g

CPSIA information can be obtained
at www.ICGtesting.com
Printed in the USA
BVHW011619120721
611731BV00010B/422